You Can Ask The Universe Anything!

Learn How to Tap Into the Infinite Field of Intelligence for Greater Clarity, Power & Insight

Michael Hetherington
BHlthSci, TCM, Yoga

First Published 2016
Mind Heart Publishing

Australia

By law this work is protected by copyright and therefore no one is permitted to copy, broadcast, transmit, show or play in public, adapt or change in any way the content of this book for any other purpose whatsoever without the prior written permission from Michael Hetherington or Mind Heart Publishing.

Disclaimer
All material in this book is provided for your information only and may not be construed as medical advice or instruction. No action or inaction should be taken based solely on the contents of this information; instead, readers should consult appropriate health professionals on any matter relating to their health and well-being.

The information and opinions expressed here are believed to be accurate, based on the best judgment available to the authors, and readers who fail to consult with appropriate health authorities assume the risk of any injuries. The publisher is not responsible for errors or omissions.

Sign up for the author's New Releases mailing list and get a free copy of *The Yin & Yang Lifestyle Guide*

www.michaelhetherington.com.au/freebook

About the Author

Michael Hetherington is a qualified acupuncturist, lecturer in Oriental medicine and yoga teacher from Brisbane, Australia. He has a keen interest in mind-body medicine, yoga nidra and Buddhist meditation. Inspired by the teachings of many, he has learned that a light-hearted, joyful approach to life serves best.

www.michaelhetherington.com.au

Other Titles by Author:

The Art of Self Muscle Testing
Learn how to access the human energy field for information

The Art of Self Adjusting
Learn how to stretch and make adjustments to the spine

EFT Through the Chakras
Work with EFT to clear the Chakras one by one

The Complete Book of Oriental Yoga
A journey into the 5 elements and yoga for the seasons

How to Do Restorative Yoga
Learn the art of a gentle yoga practice for deep relaxation

Increasing Internal Energy
Building energy from within to enhance daily life and strengthen our yoga practice

This book is a follow on from another book *The Art of Self Muscle Testing* by the same author.

It is not necessary to have read *The Art of Self Muscle Testing* before reading this book, however, it may be helpful and therefore recommended.

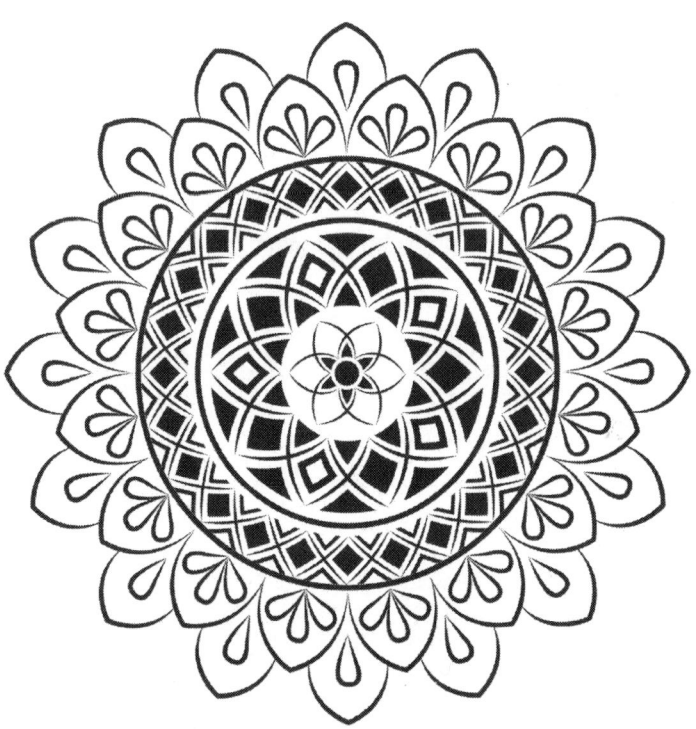

Table of Contents

INTRODUCTION	10
USE OF TERMS	13
WHY TEACH THIS?	14
EXPANDING THE PLAYING FIELD	18
HOW TO TELL IF YOU ARE READY TO ASK THE UNIVERSE ANYTHING?	29
WHEN IS IT NOT SUITABLE?	30
ASKING FOR HELP	31
HOW DO I RECOGNIZE IT?	32
THE REQUIRED CONDITIONS	37
SETTING UP PROTOCOL FOR ASKING AND RECEIVING	42
ASKING THE UNIVERSE ANYTHING	49
FINER DETAILS AND OTHER THINGS TO CONSIDER	53
HOW TO USE PERCENTAGES IN QUESTIONING TO GAIN FURTHER CLARITY	56
SUMMARY OF THE SWAY TESTING METHOD	58
THE HEART IS A NAVIGATION COMPASS	60
ESTABLISHING A RELATIONSHIP WITH THE FIELD	65
TROUBLESHOOTING – HOW AND WHY ASKING AND RECEIVING CAN BECOME INACCURATE	70
CONCLUSION	74

*At the center of your being
you have the answer;
you know who you are
and you know what you want.*

- Lao Tzu

Prologue

Before we embark on this journey together, let us verify the words and energy of this book. Let us see if these words are indeed helpful, clear and true to your heart. And if they do ring true and feel good to you, then let's embark on this journey. However, if not, it's for another time perhaps.

Let us find out.

I want you to spend a moment with this book in your hand, and/or your field of vision. Notice how you feel inside.

Take a moment.

Are you drawn forward towards it? Like a magnet, or do you feel repelled by it? In other words, do you feel yourself moving towards it, or away from it, energetically?

Do these words travel easily into your eyes and swim down to touch your heart, or are they jagged, hard to follow and hard to swallow?

If you are moving towards it and these words flow into you with ease, then yes, let's journey together. However, if you feel repelled, then likely this book is not for you – and that's ok too!

Another time perhaps.

Let us save some of your precious time and energy.

I will go into more details as to what this all means in the pages of this book. However, I just want to get us started on the right foot. There is an easy way to recognize if something will be helpful and supportive to you, just as it is easy to tell if the opposite is also true.

This is what this book is primarily about.

We will be looking, feeling and sensing into ways that will help lead us closer to clarity and truth.

As we travel through the words of this book together, I want you to check with yourself every now and then and ask,
"Does this feel true?"

If we can practice this within the pages of this book, it will be much easier to take that practice into our daily lives. One of the goals of this book is that we want life to become much clearer and obvious as to which is true and that what is… literally, nonsense. The sooner we can detect its true or nonsense quality, the better we can navigate and move onwards with much more energy, ease, and grace.

So if you are still here with me, then you feel some truth in these words and in this book already. If that is the case, then let us begin.

Introduction

Imagine if you could ask any question imaginable and receive an answer direct from the universe itself. Imagine if we could know in an instant whether something was true or not true. How much time and energy would we save by not having to "try and work it out"? What if we could just know and be done with it?

How much more space, ease and fun could things be?

When the right conditions are present and when the question being asked is without bias, yes, you can ask the universe anything!

Just picture for a moment, the universe as a giant, electromagnetic field that contains all information and knowledge of all time, complete and unending. It is made up of light, magnetism, pure vibration and a host of other elements we do not yet understand on the mental level. It is like a very complex nervous system for the entire universe. Imagine that this giant electromagnetic field is also intelligent beyond measure and fully self-aware.

This super intelligent, giant electromagnetic field is actually the field of consciousness itself, a super consciousness if you like. And what if I was to say that you can have a personal relationship with this field of consciousness, to develop a friendship with this consciousness, and be able to access all the information contained within it whenever one felt inspired to do so. Yet, what if I was to also say that not everyone can access this field of information because not everyone is 'switched on' to this level of awareness or has established a relationship with this field of consciousness.

I don't claim that this is any great secret. I don't claim of a singular method or a unique or new understanding. All I say here is that I have uncovered (alongside many others) an easy way to confirm what the mystics have been saying all along. The great teachers speak of things so far beyond the common level of consciousness that it is hard to understand and apply to one's everyday life.

What I outline in this book is a simple method, a set of techniques that helps us to "switch on" and helps us to establish an open communication channel with the field of consciousness where we can confirm certain truths for ourselves. The confirmation of certain truths will help us navigate through the trials of life for the benefit of oneself and ultimately for the benefit of all beings.

I was originally moved to write this book because I see so many people stumbling in the dark, stumbling through life with so much uncertainty and doubt in their minds. I know because I was there too, not too long ago. I hope to bring greater clarity, direction and inspiration to those who are open to receive it.

This book is a natural progression from a previous book I have written titled "The Art of Self Muscle Testing." In that book, I explored and described how to do self-muscle testing to help identify stressors in one's daily life and what you can do about it. That book is largely focused on the development of self-focused therapeutic applications of which are incredibly helpful.

However, in this book I will embark on a journey that goes further than just self-testing for therapeutic application, and focus more on how we can work directly with the field of consciousness itself, the nervous system of the universe, and be able to ask it questions and gain insight into how to most effectively live on the path of "the highest good." In this book, and with this approach, we will be moving away from the common self-help teaching of focusing on *what I want* and instead clarifying *what the universe wants*. From this re-adjusting of focus, new world and possibilities open up as we embark on the path of aligning with the highest good on all levels, which only acts to benefit others as well as oneself.

The primary reason I have embarked on this book is because the field of consciousness has given me permission to do so and is guiding my words. Therefore, this book serves as a type of transmission, a message to you from the greater field of consciousness itself. It wishes you to awaken to the truth of who you really are and to show you the way to real peace and real happiness within your heart.

This book aims to explain, in detail how to 'switch on,' how to adjust one's life so that one can readily talk to this field, and how to establish a loving connection with the field of consciousness. The ultimate purpose is to bring greater clarity, truth, love and understanding to the world for all beings to benefit.

Awaken!

Use of Terms

Throughout this book, I use a variety of terms that may be new to your vocabulary, or I may be presenting with slightly different meanings. Therefore, to help clarify the lessons in this book let's look at some of the terms commonly used.

Higher intelligence, higher power, higher self, truth, intelligent life force, the field of consciousness, the pure Self, Christ consciousness, the mind of God, the Tao, the quantum field, the Spirit - all of these terms are used interchangeably and are attempting to describe the same phenomenon. They are all pointing and descriptive words to help describe an intelligence that is greater than the sense of the individual "I".

I tend to steer away from using words such as God, love and enlightenment because these words for most of us, have been tarnished and distorted via their ongoing use in the various religious traditions. Therefore, a more modernized use of terms and terminology I have found may help serve us better in describing the various states of consciousness.

Why Teach This?

It has been becoming more and more obvious that the more people are aware of such a potential, the better it is for all. In my own journey, firstly being presented that such an idea was even possible instantly began to shift the way I perceived the world and myself in it. And, over time, with the help of the asking and receiving method, I had never felt so supported and guided than ever before. It is through that ongoing sense of support and guidance that I come to write books such as this one. To share and spread information that aids in the expansion of consciousness and perhaps more importantly, how to develop a loving and caring relationship with the pure Self or the God-like force in the universe.

With huge jumps in education, knowledge, science and technology over the past 30 years, we are moving into a new space and understanding where science, technology, and spirit can intertwine. That is not to say that all of science or technology will completely merge with spirituality, but rather some specialized fields within science are merging with technology and spiritual information. The quantum paradigm is one such example of where spirit and science can merge. The internet is an example of how technology is currently beginning to replicate the fundamentals of how information in the field of consciousness is linked and instantly accessible.

If you're looking for scientific reasoning and research to explain this phenomenon that I speak of, there isn't any, and I am not here to prove anything. All I know from my own experience, understanding and deep in my heart is that this is a very real phenomenon that I know all humans have the potential to access. The truth of it lies in the quantum field of potentiality and cannot be validated within the Newtonian scientific paradigm. It exists beyond the scientific paradigm and lays somewhere in the spiritual realm, the realm of potentiality and not of reason. It is the individual themselves that either limits themselves to this understanding, or it is for those who are awakened enough to explore this and I'm sure will find it to be true. Essentially, we will be leaning more into the field of self-experience, objective observation, and self-reflection as our primary ways of validation. In other words, *"Try it for yourself and see!"*

The method I am exploring in this book and how I came across this practice originated out of the study of applied kinesiology, also known as muscle testing. It was first really brought into the human world in the 70's via George Goodheart D.C. He discovered and created an energetic healthcare system known as 'touch for health,' which utilized modern day anatomy and physiology with the meridians and theories of Chinese medicine. You learn to uncover stressors in the body-mind matrix using 'muscle testing' to identify them. Then you can apply a corrective technique, usually by placing fingertips on various acupuncture points on the body so the identified stress can dissipate or be rebalanced.

It is a system that helps you to heal yourself and others which gives incredible results. It is rather easy to learn and is available in most countries. If you are interested, I would recommend that you enroll in a 'touch for health' course to get established with the muscle testing technique because this is one of the main techniques we use in this book to receive answers to our questions.

Dr. David Hawkins was a practicing psychiatrist around this time and came into contact with George Goodheart muscle testing system, but Dr. David Hawkins had a breakthrough realization. He realized that if you could test the energetic system of an individual, surely you could test the energetic system of the universe because we are all connected via the same system of information.

He went away and began his research with this muscle testing. He continued it for 25 years and came to some very experiential conclusions. Through his research and experimentation, he discovered that you could indeed ask the field of consciousness direct questions. Therefore, taking it beyond the one-on-one therapeutic setting and into an open dialogue with consciousness and the universe itself. And it is from the incredible work of Dr. Hawkins and my own experimentation and exploration that this book has sprung from.

The aim of this book is threefold.

1. To show you how to ask good questions and develop a personal dialogue with the higher Self & higher consciousness,
2. Explain how to use the "sway" test as the primary questioning method, and
3. Discover ways to deepen your relationship and become "friends" with the higher Self & higher consciousness

I have decided to focus on the "sway" testing method in this book as I have found it to be very effective, easy to perform and very accessible to people (it works well with absolute beginners!) rather than other techniques.

Expanding the Playing Field

Shifting the context of who, what, where, and how we see the world is essential in grasping and understanding how this process of asking and receiving answers from the universe is possible.

Every person operates within a certain context that they have built up through their belief systems, education, social conditioning and so on. Each person is operating within those "borders" set up by the context of our understanding or worldview. Every time we move into something beyond our comfort zone or study fields of knowledge less familiar to us, a re-contextualization of our worldview shifts automatically. If we pull it off, then our confidence increases and possibilities seem to expand even further in front of us, thus expanding our context even further.

When we bring a spiritual orientation into the picture the context of our experience shifts radically – perhaps more radically than other fields of knowledge or experience. Those people who choose to have faith in a higher power and have a spiritual orientation in their lives tend to have a completely different context that they operate in compared to those who do not have faith in a higher power.

Therefore, one of the primary purposes of spiritual orientation and working with methods such as the one in this book is to shift and expand our context of understanding and the context of what is possible.

Any spiritual orientation that supports the expansion of that context is generally considered helpful. Any spiritual teaching or orientation that reduces or restricts the field of context is not supportive of human development and hence, is not true spirituality.

In my previous book, "the Art of Self Muscle Testing", I was speaking mainly in regard to the context of the individual and how their individual energy field responds to the immediate environment. This approach is very useful in therapeutic settings and applications. In this book, however, I am expanding the context far further than the individual and attempting to present a context that is potentially infinite and inclusive of all beings, including the individual. We are moving away from identifying me as the center of the universe, and instead moving into the space where all is the center of the universe and my individual body and individual soul is a spark within the field of endless of sparks.

The characteristics outlined in the following pages are to help us to become more familiar with the qualities of this higher Self. It is also aimed at helping us identify it when we come into contact with it, or even when we enter its vicinity. These characteristics are universal in nature and are not restricted to a particular caste, race or religion; all human beings have access to it. The more we can acknowledge and recognize its presence in our lives, the more we can develop an ongoing relationship with it.

1. It works on the level of *essence*

One of the reasons asking and receiving from the higher realms works so well is because we are essentially testing the essence or the core vibration of things. All things, all forms have a vibrational essence, undertone or "backbone" to them. In fact, all forms and things were just an energy essence long before they became forms. Therefore, we can say that all things, form and formless, have a vibrational essence.

One of the greatest obstacles and cause of confusion for most humans is that they focus on the forms and not the essence of things. Simply put, we get tricked by the "look" of it.

Learning to read the "vibe" of things, regardless of the "look" greatly enhances one's ability to make better decisions while also removing a lot of worry and stress from our lives. The thing is, we all know how to do this already. We intuitively sense and feel the essence of things very quickly, yet we tend to ignore it or override it with our mind/ego complex.

A general principle is that all things either have an upbeat, pleasant nature to them or a downtrodden, needy, heavy nature to them regardless of how they look. The key thing is to let yourself feel it, rather than over think it or get caught up on how it "looks." In other words, go with your first gut feelings. While this is not 100% accurate all the time, it depends on the person of course, likely to be around the 70% mark as far as detecting the truth of things. And once you go through this book and learn how to do the "sway" test and develop a dialogue with the field of consciousness, you'll be more likely in the 90% accurate vicinity for detecting the essence of things.

Therefore, one of the most profound and helpful skills to learn and develop is the ability to sense the essence of things. The good news is that we already know how to do it; we just have to get out of our own way!

There are two main obstacles to developing this sense in a greater capacity. One is the ego/mind complex as mentioned previously. This involves our conditioning, memories and ego-identified preferences which are all triggered when we "over think" it. Essence is sensed only in the here and now. It is in "now" time only. As soon as you go to the mind, we leave here and now and go into the ego-complex. And because we have left the here and now, we have also lost connection with the clarity of sensing the essence.

The 2nd major obstacle that many people face is that they exist in the context of survival mode only. Survival mode is essentially the animal nature of being human. It is not bad or good; it was and still is just a part of our evolutionary process. The limitation it offers, however, is that our capacity for growth and expansion is very limited. The animal nature is only concerned with basic functions or survival, and therefore, all the potentials of other capacities and gifts of being human are left untouched. At the animal nature of the human being we have only access to basic fields of information; we tend to call them "instincts" at this level. We can detect if things are a threat to our survival, if they are helpful to our survival or if they are neutral and carry no threat or support. Essentially, these basic "instincts" are what provide us with the initial and basic skills of detecting the essence of things.

However, when we go beyond the basic functions of animal "instincts" we are able to sense a larger variety of essences, which brings more depth, color and beauty to the human experience. We can detect things such as kindness, lovingness, creativity, genius, intelligence and so on. There is a larger field of expression, sophistication, and experience that opens up to us, which naturally awakens a higher potential in the human being.

The good news is that there has been no better time in human history and no better opportunity than to keep moving beyond the basic animal nature of our makeup. While lands riddled with war, famine and lack of education do act to keep us in such an animal nature mode, the world and human nature itself, believe it or not, is creating more opportunities to move beyond it.

The more humans that move out of the basic animal nature and into the higher potentials of the human being, the greater the ability of humanity as a whole to sense the higher "essence" of things. And because of this higher capacity to sense the essence or truth of things, it will naturally burn away those things which are not supportive, healthy or true. This alignment with higher truths will play out in ways that support all of life, from the individual to the animals, planet and the universe itself.

To summarize, the steps for developing the ability to sense "*essence*" are:

1. If possible, remove or avoid situations that trigger the animal nature function. E.g War, violence, guns, aggressive music, movies and media with a lot of violence, crime, etc. It is much easier and natural to move into the higher states of human function when the nervous system can relax and register that it is in a "safe" environment.

2. Practice feeling the "vibe" of things rather than making decisions based on the "look" of it. This means giving everyone a "chance" regardless of how they look. I have found that it's the ones that you don't expect to offer many of the greatest gems of wisdom and insight.

3. Practice being in the present moment and feeling and sensing in real time – the more you think about it, the further away from being able to feel it, you will go. Usually, the feeling of things is experienced in the core of the torso around the belly and heart areas in particular. Practice "checking in" with this space a number of times throughout the day.

4. If unsure or confused and can't shake it, sleep on it. Then soon after you wake, what is the first feeling you get on it when you revisit it with your attention?

Consider your ability to sense the essence of things as having a wise inner teacher with you who is available 24/7.

2. It communicates through a language of energetic vibrations

Every question we ask is seen in the field of consciousness not as English or French in the field but of an energetic, vibrational, electrical, print – in other words – a pulse of vibrational energy. It reads our questions and intentions as energetic prints through the field. It then interprets the energetic print as our intention or question (the essence) and responds as a surge of energy which we interpret as a "yes" or "no." Some people can receive more information beyond the "yes" or "no" such as flashes of images or colors or sounds, yet the method we are focusing on in this book is a simple yes or no – which is, and can easily be enough to get clarity to the questions we ask.

The language of the field is very sophisticated, and it is often difficult for humans to translate it into something of value or meaning that can be understood. It is received more so on the feeling level than the mental level. However, humans are getting increasingly clever at translating feeling level vibrations to mental level understanding.

To simplify the process of communication and receiving understandable responses from the field of consciousness itself, we will be working on the level of "yes" and "no" responses only.

What we are receiving as a "yes" is essentially an instantaneous pulse of pure vibration coming from deep within. When that harmonic vibration intensifies enough to affect our personal energy field, it naturally boosts it with a "shot" of "Qi" or universal life force energy.

"No" on the other hand expresses itself as an instantaneous pulse of inharmonic vibration. It is unsteady and wavering in its structure, and when it becomes charged enough to influence our personal energy field it "weakens" us a little – just momentarily.

Another important point to mention here is that to every question that is asked it also generates an answer (energetic print) somewhere in the universe at that exact moment. This is due to the law of creative potential. It is not possible to create a question without an answer also being created – for a question would not be a question unless an answer too existed. You see, questions need answers to exist and so answers need questions to exist too. Therefore, it may be comforting to know that to every question you ask, there is an answer that has been created too. It is also worth mentioning here that answers don't always come through as being verbal or linguistically supportive in nature. They can come in many forms, such as an understanding, a vision, a dream, a feeling or even a random movement of the body may prove to be a suitable answer.

When we learn to focus on the essence or vibration of things, we will find that even when different people use the same words and ask exactly the same questions, they will often receive very different answers. This is a direct result of the field responding to the essence and vibration of that person and their question and not to the superficial words themselves. Therefore, that is why we must ask and receive the answers ourselves, to experience it ourselves, rather than take on other people's answers and insights as our own. At various stages of the journey and as we move through different states of consciousness, the questions and answers will naturally change also.

Time to check in with yourself now –
Do these words feel true?

Is this closer to truth?

3. It does not seek to control

When opening ourselves up to the potential of asking and receiving questions from the universe, it's important to understand that the field we are accessing is not trying to control us in any way.

Free will still exists, and it understands that it is up to us what we do with the information we receive. These higher states of consciousness are always present in us and are ready to guide us, yet they do not use any force or use coercion to win their way. The field is patient and compassionate, allowing us to experience it for ourselves and come to our own realization of its presence and power.

Later on, as our consciousness becomes more and more open to its presence, there is a space we come to where it feels natural to "let go" and "allow" the energy of this higher state consciousness to move through us unhindered. This "allowing" process allows for these higher states and vibration of energy to move through our mind-body field, burning away all the old and limiting patterns and habits. This can trigger a "healing crises" which is simply the process of the old ego patterns being burnt away as the person in question comes to see the world and themselves with new eyes.

As we continue to do this and pass through the "healing crises" stages, eventually things begin to smooth out and calm down. As things calm down, life takes on a pace of much less effort, strain, worry or tension. There opens up, even more, allowing and trust to which our behaviors become guided with more ease and grace by something beyond the self. Other qualities of this space include more joy, playfulness, and wisdom.

4. Will help you to love (yourself) more

Another quality of experiencing this asking and questioning process is that it will always be in the direction of helping to increase the love for oneself and towards others. It will never offer answers that encourage anything away from love and clarity.

Love, the word itself, is often misunderstood to be an emotion, a feeling or a particular expression of behavior. However, real love has little to do with emotions and behaviors and has more to do with a way of being.

When you add the term *unconditional* to the word love, we are talking about love as "a one-way street." It requires no reason or recognition for it is complete in itself. Emotional love is often a "2-way street," meaning it requires some particular behavior or expression from another person or outside influence to be able to "love" them back.

Some people think they are practicing "unconditional love" yet they often feel drained or feel like it's a lot of work to keep it up. This is not true unconditional love because unconditional love does not come from the person; it comes through them from the field and is therefore not draining upon their personal energy. If we feel drained, or like something is a lot of effort, it's coming from our own ego/mind construct and not the higher Self. One way to overcome this "efforting" is to stop trying to do unconditional love and just relax into it. Give up the idea you need a reason to love someone or something. Give up the idea you need to achieve something or do something before you can love yourself… Is existence not enough? Allow yourself to bathe in this sense of appreciation without any effort, trying, expectation or movement.

When asking questions to the higher Self, it will only respond in a way that brings us closer to truth, clarity and the energy of unconditional love – so much so that on the mental or rational level it is likely that we will not understand some of the answers we receive, at first.

We have to take into account that we are asking a "super" intelligent system questions and that the answers we will sometimes receive will make little sense. This can often lead us to discard the responses we receive due to their perplexing nature. However, as we develop an ongoing "friendly" and trusting relationship with it, we will increasingly follow its revelations without much hesitation. And is often the case, in future times when we reflect back upon some answers, there will be a better understanding and sense of clarity as to those answers we received.

How to Tell if You Are Ready to Ask the Universe Anything?

If you are even drawn to this book, and indeed still reading, then it is a strong indicator that you are ready to do the question and answer process.

It is also likely that you have already been working on developing your sensitivity to this type of exploration, or you are inherently attuned to the subtle energies of the universe that I speak of – all of this providing you with an ideal, and heightened capacity to receive clear and accurate answers.

People who are considered "sensitive" or "empaths" are particularly receptive to this type of work. Being sensitive must be seen as a gift rather than a curse – yet to do so, those who are sensitive in such a way will need to make some effort to position themselves into occupations where they can thrive and continue to develop their "power." Such people are generally suited to the fields of healers, artists, visionaries, academics and agriculturists.

When is it NOT Suitable?

There are some times in our lives where the asking and receiving process is not ideal or not appropriate. If we are in the middle of an intense emotional upheaval; if we are very tired, upset, or under the influence of drugs or alcohol, it is not suitable to test. Nothing will stop you from trying, but the results are unlikely to be clear and reliable.

In such states, it is often best to wait and let the storm pass before attempting to test again. Often simply going to sleep allows the storm to pass and for the body-mind to reset.

Another thing to be aware of is the more emotionally invested we are in a question; the harder it is to receive clear answers because there is "bias" present. I explore this more in a later chapter where we talk about creating the right conditions for testing. In such instances, it can be a good idea to get a friend or colleague to test it for you as they will be a lot less invested in it than you.

Asking for Help

The first step in accessing higher intelligence and higher power, whether you are testing or just seeking extra support in any endeavor, is to simply ask for it.

And in asking for its support, you are acknowledging its existence also. Therefore, both acknowledgment as well as the act of asking for support, opening a dialogue with it, is all that is needed to begin working with it.

If we do not acknowledge its existence, then how can we access it? We, therefore, cut ourselves off from it through the use of exercising our own will to remove it from our awareness and attention.

This is not about believing in something; it is about recognizing, experiencing and knowing something to be true or not. This is where we want to go. Knowing and experiencing hold much more power than a belief because belief is associated with our mental level only, whereas knowing and experiencing is associated with the whole sense of one's being.

How Do I Recognize It?

In this chapter, I will talk more about how to recognize when you are in clear connection with the higher Self. The purpose being that the more you get familiar with it, the easier and more natural it will be for you to connect to it.

Whenever you are in direct contact with the higher Self-expression, you feel clear, calm, alert and joyful for no particular reason. It presents itself whenever we are not caught up in "the story". The story is the drama and timeline of events we use to justify who we think we are and why we are the way we are. It's the continuous pattern of moving back into the past and "the story" through the use of the facilities of the mind. When you are aligned with the higher Self, there is no story. The mind is still there, yet it is insignificant and "over to the side" to one's awareness. Plain and simple. When you are connected with higher Self, you are just here, present, alive and receptive.

While it can be helpful every now and then to reflect on the past for healing, growth, and even humor, generally, the more we talk about it, think about it, and generally dive deeper into the story, the further we go away from the higher Self. One of the main points here is if you want to be more in touch with the higher Self, focus your point of attention on the unfolding of life as it is happening now. It can be as simple as watching your breath, feeling into your body, or just watch life happening around you without labeling it. The more you withdraw your attention from "the story" and place it in the presence of the higher Self, the more the story and all the anxiety and stress that comes along with it falls away.

There is often other feelings involved, such as fun, playfulness, openness, vibrancy; however, these types of feelings can change according to the particular person and their unique vibrational makeup. For example, one person may easily move into states of fun & expressive bodily movement as their higher self-expression, yet another would more easily slip into states of being more cheeky and humorous. However, while personalities can differ slightly in their higher self-expressions, there will always be an undertone of feeling clear, vibrant and generally joyful.

Excitement is one feeling that is often associated with the higher states of self; however, it is not always the case. Excitement has many different expressions and can be triggered for different reasons. Some excitement can be triggered by adrenaline-type sports, while other states that we would call excitement could be triggered from simply by the thought of seeing someone we love again. These two examples offer us completely two different expressions of excitement, so it's important to understand the difference.

Generally, excitement is a positive experience; however, it is unsustainable. Why? Because, in most cases, we have associated excitement to the adrenaline physiological responses, and adrenaline is an energy source that is
1. Unsustainable
2. Comes from the lower, animal mind and is not rooted in the higher self

Therefore, the excitement that is tied to the adrenal response is not an ideal feeling to associate with the higher self or higher states of consciousness. Other, yet somewhat similar expressions to excitement can be states of joy. And joy, unlike excitement, is sustainable.

When we work with our higher self, our physiology, and our physical bodies begin to change. And the more we rest or sit in the states of the higher self, the more our physiology starts to organize into a new state of being.

For example, different parts of the brain, such as those parts responsible for higher states of consciousness, cognitive thinking, information processing, and language become more activated and stable. Those parts of the brain linked to reactive, animal, fight or flight responses increasingly "deactivate" as they are less and less needed or required. The heart rate also begins to change its rhythms to a more regular, steady and slower rate, as the person accesses higher levels of consciousness. Breathing becomes more efficient as the body is generally more relaxed. Organs and tissues repair with greater ease and effectiveness. There is a host of physiological changes, too many to go into any great detail here simply due to the body and mind moving into higher states of consciousness and the slow deactivation, and less dependence on the "fight or flight" animal-like nature responses.

Physiological changes can become so profound that common "normal" reactions become obsolete or minimized. For an extreme example, when higher functions and physiological systems are established, things like drugs, alcohol, and sugar have little to no effect on the system. This is because they are operating in an energy field that gains its energy and information from the higher self and therefore is not easily influenced or affected by the dense physical reactions of the world.

A quick exercise to recognize the state and feeling of your higher self:

1. Close your eyes and think back to a memory when you felt most alive and joyful.
   Visualize yourself in front of you now.
   See yourself smiling with joy.
2. Allow the feeling of that joy from that experience to come into your body now.
   Breathe it in.
3. Now, what are the qualities of this state?
   Can you describe them? E.g. Joyful, alive, fun, etc.

These qualities you are naming are likely to be the state of your higher self.

It is important to know and understand that you can put yourself in this state at any time, and it's available always. The easiest way is to practice moving into the "feeling" of this higher state. Thoughts are helpful but "feelings" are much stronger in power. The more you practice the "feeling" state of your higher self, the more present it becomes in your day-to-day experience and the easier it is to ask the universe anything!

Question:
When you feel most alive and clear, what qualities do you embody?

Are you humorous? Fun? Witty? Creative? Energetic?

Your answers will give you insight into what your natural, higher Self is and feels like.

The Required Conditions

In the previous chapters, we have spent some time exploring the various qualities of the field of consciousness. And so now that those foundations are in place, it's now time to move into the more practical elements – bringing us more and more into the space of experiential understanding.

Certain conditions or prerequisites need to be in place before accurate feedback from the questioning process can be attained. This is especially true when you are new to the process. When the conditions and prerequisites are not in place, the answers tend to come back inaccurate, unclear and inconsistent.

There are 5 primary prerequisites that need to be in place before accurate testing can begin. They are:

1. Spiritual orientation
2. Integrity – to be sincere
3. Non-bias questioning
4. Reduce or avoid low-energy environments
5. Be "switched on."

1. Spiritual orientation
For a person to be able to ask and communicate clearly with the universe, they will need to have some kind of spiritual orientation in their life. Generally, those people who follow a faith are

spiritually inclined or are agnostic will be able to access the answers given by the universal force.

Those who have no spiritual orientation running through their lives follow atheism or have no faith in a higher power will not have easy access offered by the universal force. This is because due to the absence of acknowledgment they automatically cut themselves off from accessing it. Without acknowledgment, there can be no conscious awareness.

Having a spiritual orientation also has nothing to do with how many times one goes to Church or to the temple, or how much yoga practice one does. As well as that, having a spiritual orientation is not about "believing" in something. True spiritual orientation is about *sensing, knowing* and *experiencing* some kind of higher intelligence operating in their lives and acknowledging its presence.

This is not to say that those without a spiritual orientation are cut off from it entirely. For it is always present and waiting, infinitely patient and doesn't want anything from us, so it's not going to try and trick us or punish us in any way.

Faith and trust are also qualities that are present in those who have spiritual orientation. Faith and trust often manifest in a person who is very calm, relaxed and content regardless of their outside circumstances. This is because they feel "secure" in their heart and in the power of the higher Self.

2. Integrity – to be sincere
Integrity comes out of valuing life and supporting it in any form it's expressed. It involves feeling into and establishing a value system that is based on virtue, respect for life in all its expressions and compassion.

Integrity means taking responsibility for your life and not projecting and blaming our misfortune on others, governments, the economy, etc. Integrity is an awareness that you are your own master and guru and that how you respond, react and behave is entirely up to you.

It also implies sincerity. When we are sincere in our seeking for answers and in the growth and development of true understanding, we express sincerity. If we are not sincere in our asking and receiving it is unlikely to produce any real obvious or clear answers because it knows that we are not really interested in the answers.

3. Non-bias questioning

This is a big one and one that often destabilizes our ability to receive clear answers. Non-bias questioning means that we don't have an invested interest in the outcome when we ask questions. This can be a hard practice to master because naturally, we are very interested in many of the answers on a personal level.

Before asking and testing, it's important to see and witness how emotionally "charged up" you are around the issue. If you feel strongly emotional around the issue, you're unlikely to receive a clear answer.

There are a few strategies to get around it:

1. Practice "Stepping back" and detaching yourself from yourself and the outcome. It's about asking and receiving your answers in a purely, objective space. Not always easy, yet when you do this successfully, you will get a clear answer.
2.

Practices like Vipassana meditation are really helpful for "stepping back" and just watching without the emotional involvement.

3. Get a friend or 3rd party who can do the asking and testing method (e.g. the sway test) to do it for you. It is always easier to test for other people, especially those whom you do not know well than it is to test for yourself.

4. Don't test it. Either let it go this time around or try sleeping on it and trying again when you're less "involved" in the outcome.

4. Reduce or avoid testing in a low-level consciousness environments

This simply means that the space you wish to do the testing and to encourage clear and accurate results needs to be a quiet, clean, airy and nicely lit. Having plants in the space also assists with keeping our energy field circulating easily.

These kinds of environments support the testing process because they allow for clarity and higher vibrations to be present. It is not always necessary to be so considerate of space, for eventually people who build up their skills with such a process can literally test in any location. However, for beginners and people looking to develop these skills, using a good environment will help establish a clearer connection and response.

5. To be "switched on"

This simply means that the person testing has a clear head and feels suitable and willing to test. If you feel foggy-headed, really tired, dehydrated or have a body full of aches and pains, then this is not a "Switched on" state. There are a few things you can do practically to support the body and mind to be in a more ready "switched on" state. I discuss these techniques in greater detail in my previous book, "the art of self-muscle testing"; however, I will summarize them here.

1. Have a sip of pure, clean water.
2. Rub acupressure point Kid 27 for 15 seconds.
3. Rub just below the belly button and lower back for 15 seconds.
4. Stand up straight, and breathe in through the nose.
5. Let go of thinkingness for a moment and see if you feel clear.
6. If you feel clear you are likely in a "switched on" state, so conduct the testing. If you don't feel clear, you can try rubbing the points again to "recheck" yourself. If you're not clear at all, better wait for another time.

Setting Up Protocol for Asking and Receiving

For this book, I want to discuss and describe primarily the "Sway" testing method. After having shown and taught some testing methods over many years, I have found the "Sway" testing method to be most effective and easiest for people to pick up, especially at the beginning.

I have taught and shown the sway testing method in a variety of formal and non-formal settings and with a large variety of people. I have taught it to massage students in classrooms, to patients in clinic, to friends in restaurants and even to strangers in bars (that's what you get for asking me what it is that I do). And every time I have taught it, it has worked 99.9% of the time.

The .1% that the sway test doesn't seem to work is usually experienced in older individuals whose bodies tend to be in an incredibly stiff state and have been for a long period. The stiffness is due to ongoing illness, recent surgeries, pains in the body and prolonged periods of immobility. The stiffening of the tissues seems to impede the ability of the energy to flow and move easily through the system, therefore distorting the ability to sense the sway. Another factor here that can impede the sway test with this individual is that their "center of gravity" is out of balance. In other words, they have difficulty standing in a relaxed, balanced, natural position as the body is continuously leaning into an off-center position making it incredibly difficult to use the sway method. Therefore, keep these things in mind when working with the sway test on yourself as well as on others.

The sway testing method is the easiest way to get started and develop our sensitivities to our energy field and the asking and receiving process. I want to emphasize that the sway testing method itself is just a tool, and is therefore just a means to an end.

Let's now go through and explain the sway testing method so that you can get familiar with it and then, I will explain how it works.

The Simple "Yes" and "No" Sway Test

The yes and no test is a test that I recommend everyone to do at the beginning to help them get a "sense" of what the answers feel as they send a wave of energy through the body. For there is a definitive "wave" of energy that moves through the body whenever we say yes or no (all the time, we just don't notice its subtlety). To get a clearer sense of it and notice it more easily, it helps to stand up into a natural position and relax the body.

Ok, so this is how we do it…

Standing

1. The sway test simply refers to a test that involves a person standing with feet shoulder width apart, knees just off lock,

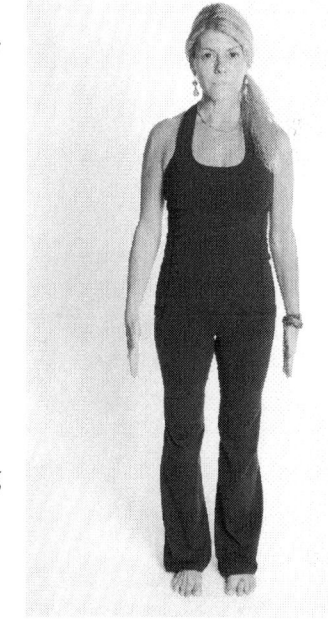

shoulders and arms relaxed. The person should be standing in a "neutral", relaxed position.

2. First, we want to test "yes". We do this by saying the word out loud, **repeatedly** (yes, yes, yes, yes) and applying our attention to the word and the vibration of the word.

3. Then notice and observe what happens to the body. (There will be a natural swaying motion – which way does it sway? If everything is working properly, the body will sway forward.)

4. Next, we want to test "no". We do this by saying the work out loud, **repeatedly** (no, no, no, no) and applying our attention to the word and the vibration of the word. (Again, the body will want to sway in a particular direction – which way does it sway? If everything is working properly, the body will sway backward.)

(Pictures on next page..)

(NO!)　　　　　　　(YES!)

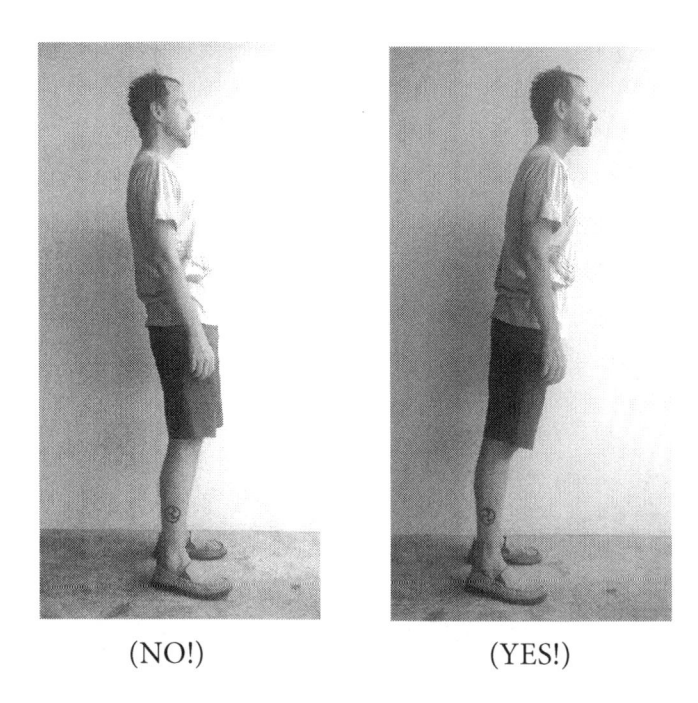

When we feel the wave of energy move through us (**yes = forward, no = backward**) and as it becomes more and more obvious, it's time to move to the next test.

The True and False Statement Test

This is the second test I would recommend before moving onto the big questions. This is a way to experience for ourselves whenever we lie or say something that is not "true" to our hearts, which will cause us to move backward. However, when we tell the truth and say things that support our heart, we will always move forward towards it. (This is essentially a polygraph test!)

1. The sway test simply refers to a test that involves a person standing with feet shoulder width apart, knees just off-lock, shoulders and arms relaxed. The person should be standing in a "neutral," relaxed position.

5. First, we want to test the "truth". We do this by saying, "My name is……." out loud, **repeatedly** and focusing our attention on the word and the vibration of the word.

   Notice and observe what happens to the body. (There will be a natural swaying motion – which way does it sway? If everything is working properly, the body will sway forward).

6. Next, we want to test a "lie". We do this by saying, "my name is [false name]" out loud, **repeatedly** and focusing our attention on the word and the vibration.

   Again, the body will want to sway in a particular direction. (Which way does it sway? If everything is working properly, the body will sway backward.)

You can try different questions if you like to test it out for yourself. It is best to stick to simple questions here, and at the beginning of every session, as we need to train ourselves to get used to the feeling and sensitivity of the responses. The bigger questions come later when we have established a clear question and response from the field.

Some examples of simple true and false questions are:

"I am ....years old."
"I am from ….."
"…… is my favorite food."

Getting Grounded & Clear

This is an added practice which I find very powerful at grounding our energies and getting really clear and stable. We simply say these sentences, one at a time, repeatedly, and see if we sway forward or backward on each statement. If we move backward on any of them just stop for a second, take a breath and focus on your feet and visualize a light-emanating rod in the core of your body and your being. As a complementary practice, I have also found that it helps to look at an image or statue of the Buddha or some saintly being.

After a moment of taking a good breath and using the visuals, test the statement again.

When you go forward on all of these statements, you will feel very clear and "switched on."

The grounding process to finish set up
1. **I am grounded**
2. **I am integrated**
3. **I am centered**
4. **I have permission to ask**

Asking for permission is always a good idea before getting into some of the heavy questions. Sometimes, it may not be necessary or beneficial for us to know the answers to the questions we seek, or it simply may not be the right time to know. Therefore, we may get a sway backward ("no" response) to asking permission. Whenever we get this response, better to let it go and move on. You can change the subject of the question, and it may then say "yes." In such a case, it's ok to ask. But if you get the "no" response repeatedly during a session, stop what you're doing and go do something else – now is not the right time! Respect it. Don't push it. You can always try again tomorrow if need be.

Asking the Universe Anything

Once we have done the setup protocol and everything has come back clear and affirmed you are now ready to ask the universe anything.

In this chapter, I will provide you the practical explanation and offer a few examples of how to ask and receive answers from the higher consciousness field. The aim here is to get you familiar with the practical process and allow your consciousness to expand with the presentation of these concepts so that when we discuss more of the details and principles in the following chapters you will have a better grasp as to what they refer to.

The key to wisdom and insight is not so much in the knowing of answers but in the asking of good questions.

Before we go any further, it is important to spend some time talking about "right" and "wrong", "good" and "bad" in the context of asking the universe anything. When we work with the field, there is no such thing as right and wrong, good and bad. In the context of the field, there is only truth and clarity and the absence of those things. The absence of truth and clarity is haziness, lack of clarity, confusion, and superficial trivialities. So when we are working with the field in this way, we are essentially asking, "Is this question and answer close to the truth and clarity, which will either have a "yes" response or a "no" response."

SOME QUESTIONS TO ASK THE UNIVERSE…

Once you have completed the protocols this is how to start formulating and asking your questions:

Fundamentals:
1, Make sure you have set up the right conditions for clear testing. (E.g. checking yourself, removing bias, etc.)

2. Stand in the neutral posture.

3. Focus on the object you want to ask about and then ask your question without distraction.

"Is this …. True?"

Another example of a question would be to simply look at the object, person, book, movie, and ask.
"Is this …. True?"

3. Try to keep the questions short and clear so that you don't confuse yourself or the field. If you get distracted or start thinking about something else, the energy will shift to the new object of attention. Therefore, if you get distracted, start the process again.

4. If unclear, repeat the question 2 or 3 times, saying it out aloud.

5. Observe to see if the body moves forward or backward. Forward means "yes" and backward means "no."

Examples of subjects and questions you can ask.

Verification Process
Is this book close to truth?
Is the energy of this book close to truth?
Does this practice bring me closer to truth?
Is this movie/book/information close to truth?

Political
This politician is close to truth?
Is communism close to truth?
Is socialism close to truth?
Is democracy close to truth?

Other Life Forms
Is it necessary to know if extraterrestrials exist?
Do extraterrestrials exist?
Are all extraterrestrials the same?
Are there over 1million galaxies?
Can humans survive on other planets?
Does water exist on other planets?
Is it necessary to know?

History + Future Projections
Is it true that…happened in history? (e.g. 1932 etc.)
Was Cleopatra (or anybody in history) killed against her will?
The next economic crises (enter more details here) will occur in 5 years?

Is global warming caused by humans?
Will the planet survive regardless of what humans do?

Higher Questions of Spirit
Does God exist?
Am I on the path of my highest good?
Is everyone destined for enlightenment?
Does enlightenment exist?
I am motivated by (love, greed, lust, integrity, etc.)?
Jesus was a real man who walked the earth 2000 years ago?
Is it necessary for me to know?

Significant People in Human History
Is Mahatma Gandhi close to truth?
Is Carl Marx close to truth?
Is Einstein close to truth?
Is Barack Obama close to truth?

Finer Details and Other Things to Consider

1. Generally, depending on the person, and especially when you are new to this, you have about **10-15 minute open window to ask your questions**. After that time, too many questions and too many answers tend to overwhelm and confuse the nervous system. When you start feeling a bit overwhelmed, unclear or are struggling to find new questions to ask, it's time to take a break.

2. Nothing in the future is absolutely certain; there are only probabilities based on the current trajectory of energy flow. Future answers are based on high likelihoods rather than absolutes.

3. When you get multiple "yes" to questions that seem to contradict, break it down into percentages. (Discussed in more detail in next section)

4. In your questioning, use time scales and detail to gain clearer insight. However, in saying that, keep the questions as short and as less wordy as possible.

5. Due to the nature of this process, we may receive answers and ask questions that we have never asked before. Therefore, sometimes, answers can be so mind-shattering that it will take some time to integrate it after the answer has come through. Depending on the person, it can take anywhere from a few days

to years to integrate a big answer into their way of seeing the world.

Politics and Testing

It continues to boggle me how so many people invest so much of their energy, time and money into debating street-level, uninformed politics.

In regards to the essence of political parties and their representatives, what you will find is that with the sway testing method you can discover whether a particular political party will be supportive to the society or not.

It can be as simple as resting your eye gaze on one of the leaders or a group of them who represent the political party and ask:
Is this party close to the truth?
Or
Is this party supportive of life?

If you go forward – Yes! They are going in such a direction.
If you go back – No! Avoid them and look into the other options.

Could it be that simple?

Yes!

Be aware that no political party or human for that matter will get everything perfect, so why do we even expect such things? Is it not good enough to know that they are going in the right direction? Those political parties and candidates that are not going in the right direction should be avoided and abandoned as soon as possible.

At higher levels of truth, when the individual attains great understanding, the need for political parties, politicians, police, armies, and governments, in general, is no longer required. Why? Because an awakened person, a person who understands the laws of the universe and man becomes self-governed. It becomes obvious what word and deed are appropriate and true. There is no longer the need to control, rehabilitate or govern anyone on how to live and cooperate in a human society because it is clear and obvious to an awakened being.

How to Use Percentages in Questioning to Gain Further Clarity

After some experience with testing and receiving answers, you will eventually come across answers that say "yes" to two or more things that may appear contradictory.

For example, you may ask
    1. Is Mahatma Gandhi close to truth
    2. Is Mother Teresa close to truth
The answer to both = "yes."

So, if we receive any "no" response, it is clear and not necessary to break it down for a "no" response simply means that it's less than 50% true and therefore not worthwhile exploring any further. It's simply best to avoid it and move on. However, with two or more "yes" responses, we can break it down further by asking a question like:

Is Mahatma Gandhi close to truth at 60%?
70?
80? Etc.
Is it above 90%? - no
Is it above 85%? - no
Is it above 82%? – yes
Is it 84% exactly? – no
Is it 83% exactly? – yes
Ok, it is 83% yes that Mahatma Gandhi is close to truth…

We can repeat the question again; however, remembering that the field is super intelligent, it knows what question you are referring to. Therefore, it is, in most cases unnecessary to repeat. However, if you break your train of thought, it will be necessary to repeat the question. (Avoid breaking your train of thought because every time you do that you shift your energy and lose the original energy print of the question).

Then, we can gain clarity on the other yes question.
Is Mother Teresa close to truth at 60%? – yes
Above 70% - yes
Above 80% – no
Above 75% - no
Above 73% - no
Is it 72% exactly? – yes

Ok, so there we have our results (just an example).

1. Mahatma Gandhi is close to truth at 83%
2. Mother Teresa is close to truth at 72%

So now you have very clear and detailed information as to what is closer to truth. Both are great and worthwhile to have around and learn from. However, Mahatma Gandhi may be able to take things a little further.

What you do with the information is entirely up to you.

Summary of the Sway Testing Method

1. Check yourself to see if you feel "switched on"

2. Do the simple "Yes" and "No" test

3. Do the Truth and False Statement test

4. When answers come back clear and accurate, you can begin to move onto the bigger questions.

5. Ask for permission to test

6. Ask your bigger questions (You usually have about a 10-15 minute window per session.)

7. If you get multiple "yes" responses, and you want more clarity, use the percentage scale to clarify the "yes" statements

8. That's it!

It's essentially up to you what you do with the information. Remember that it will never lead or encourage us to harm anything. And it is always working for our higher good. It is a normal response for many to feel slightly overwhelmed by the process, and such a situation will require a "resting" period after the testing to help integrate the new awareness into their being.

Many times it can be difficult to come up with good questions because we are not used to thinking that way. Never before have we been able to ask the universe direct questions and receive an answer almost instantly. This is the beauty and magic of connecting with and working with the infinite life force itself.

What a blessing it is!

The Heart is a Navigation Compass

In this section, we will explore another way to sense a supportive "yes" or an unsupportive "no" response. We can access it by focusing our attention on our heart space as we question.

If there was a center of the energetic field of the human being, it would be the physical heart itself. This is because the heart produces the strongest electromagnetic field in the entire body. The electrical field produced by the heart is 60 times more powerful in amplitude than the one produced in the brain. Therefore, through the phenomenon of entrainment, the brain wave patterns can be easily influenced by the pulse of the heart.

The origins of the initial electrical pulse in the heart, when we are in the womb, are still a mystery. Doctors and scientists still cannot explain how the heart begins its electrical pulse activity. Within the context of this book, we could say that the heart is the original organ from where the spirit moves through the unmanifest world, into the manifest world, with its first layer being an electrical "kick" through the physical heart – hence producing life on the physical, manifest world. Because of the heart's unique and powerful contribution to our energy field, we can use it as a guide and compass.

This requires an ability to listen to the feelings and pulses of the heart in relation to when we hold things in the mind's eye. Let's use an example so you can gain a better understanding as to what I'm talking about.

Sensing the Heart Compass

1. Ok, so first, take a moment to listen to your heart. You may be able to feel a pulse, or not; it doesn't matter. What is more important than sensing the pulse is to become aware of the chest area, and notice how it feels. Is it tight, relaxed? Do you find it easy to breathe, difficult to breathe? No need to change anything; just become aware of what's going on.

2. Now, bring someone you deeply admire and appreciate. It can be a family member, a saintly person who you hold in high regard, or a friend you care deeply for. Now, with them etched into your mind's eye, notice what's going on again in the heart (chest) area. 10-30 seconds is often enough.

3. Then, think of someone who has caused great suffering to humanity. Hitler is often an easy one to bring up as everyone knows him and can easily picture his unique mustache and Nazi uniform in our minds. Now, with him in your mind's eye, notice what's going on in your chest area. 10 -20 seconds is enough.

    What do you notice? Is it tighter or more relaxed?

4. Now, to finish, think of a candle flame. A gentle, graceful flame dancing in your mind's eye. Now, with that in mind, notice your chest area again. 10 -30 seconds is enough.

5. When ready, relax your posture and take a sip of water.

Time to reflect.

What did you notice? What were the feelings you felt when you went from a saint or family member to Hitler and then to a gentle candle flame?

If you were able to sense the shifts, then 90% of the world population would respond in a similar manner in regards to the sensations in the heart area.

* Someone highly regarded in your mind's eye would produce an open, soft, relaxed chest area.

* Hitler would produce a tightness, restriction, uncomfortableness in the chest area.

* A gentle candle flame – a gentle, easeful and relaxed chest area.

This is because it works on exactly the same principles as already mentioned in this book. Those things that support our life force and support the health and vitality of our energy field will produce a softening, open, relaxed feeling in the body's energy field, and in particular the chest area. Those things that are harmful or stressful to our energy field will produce a tightened, restricted chest area.

Just to clarify, this is when we conduct this exercise without being biased.

The more sensitive to the heart and chest area we become, the more we feel whether things are good for us or not.

We can use this awareness for making a decision or regarding any challenge we may be faced with because the heart (spirit doorway) knows more than the mind will ever know. Spirit is also connected to the future because, in the spirit realm, future and present are one and the same. So if you wish to ask things about the future, from my experience, go with the heart test.

How to use the heart compass test for making decisions:

1. First, get clear about the options you are faced with. Sometimes writing them down and putting a circle or a square mark around them helps to focus energy on the option.

2. Next, bring your full attention to one of your options. You can pull up some kind of image or scene in your mind of the option - what the environment looks like, feels like, etc.

3. Then simply notice your heart space – is it tight and restricted or open, relaxed and flowing?

4. Repeat this process with the next option. Bring an image or feeling of the option into your mind and body. Then notice the heart space – is it open and flowing or tight and relaxed..?

5. Now, after you have gone through them all. Which one or one(s) generated an open, relaxed feeling in the heart area? **That is the one to go for.**

Any option that produced tightness – throw it out.

To further confirm your findings, try the test again another day or even the next day. There could be a slight chance of being invested in the outcome and therefore become biased regarding a particular option which could give you incorrect indicators. However, if you do it a few times over a few days, the answers become increasingly clear. You will often get the feeling deep in your body and bones regarding which is the right path to take after a few days of testing.

Establishing a Relationship with the Field

The most important relationship is the one we have with ourselves, and the field itself, which in other words is our Higher Self. When we are aligned with our Higher Selves, this means that we are putting ourselves in direct contact with the field itself. This is because the field is one that is benevolent and loving, so when we focus on and develop that quality in ourselves, we naturally come closer to alignment with the field.

When there is a connection between the self and the field, everything tends to flow with grace and ease. However, if that relationship is not connected, discarded or ignored, life tends to become a real effort and struggle. Depression is the most common sign of disconnect from the self and the higher field – for when we are connected, it is not even possible to feel such things! Therefore, the more we learn to connect with, listen to and develop a loving friendship with ourselves and the field, the more aligned and empowered our daily lives will become.

This is one of the most profound relationships that will naturally take shape after an ongoing practice and establishment of processes like "energy field testing". It largely comes from the ongoing practice and fine-tuning of "checking in with the self" and asking of sincere questions. This is because, after a while of asking questions to "The field" of the universe, you naturally develop a kind of unique dialogue with it. You begin to develop an acute sense as to what the answers are to your questions as you ask them, and you even get prompted or nudged to reframe your questions at some points.

One begins to clearly feel that there is some kind of intelligent force working with one in a very direct and personal way. As I mentioned earlier, while the field tends to be mostly "impersonal" - meaning it doesn't care what your opinions are - it just delivers truths as to what is supportive of our energy and what is not. After some time developing a dialogue with it, it does begin to feel personal. At some point, you may even begin to feel a non-physical guide, light being or even an angelic presence come into your questioning process.

For example, as I write these words now, it's as if I am talking about another person who is not present. However, when I intuitively ask if they are indeed present, they are. They are fully here with me now, guiding me as I write. They are supportive of me talking about them the same way they want more of us human beings to be open and receptive to their communications. And this work, this book, is just one other way through which they can communicate.

It is indeed a "they" for it indicates that there is more than one present. I am not sure the exact numbers, but there are quite a few. The more I talk with and about them, the more they seem to gather around me adding more energy into this writing process.

How remarkable!

So the main message they wish to share with you here is that you can ask the universe anything. And while the field itself is able to respond, there are also higher dimensional beings that can work with you and guide you. They can answer via a variety of ways, but the one highlighted throughout this book is through the sway testing method, which allows us access to clear YES or NOs with our sway testing.

They also want to say that whenever we are in the presence of a higher consciousness being, whether physical or non-physical, that we do and will experience a surge or heightened sense of life force energy as it moves through us.

They want us to know and learn to recognize this for ourselves, which many of us already do, so we can use it more readily and easily when navigating our world.

We lack direct hearing and communication with higher levels of consciousness due to a number of factors. The main one being that we lack the "context" for which they can operate more easily in. If we have created our world that is of a small context, for example, where my mind is my only source of information, then we're cut off from such thing as "higher consciousness beings" as the capacity to speak to higher dimensional beings is dramatically reduced because we do not even acknowledge that they exist. If we were to allow our contextual framework to be far-reaching, to be more inclusive of abstract ideas and concepts, then naturally, we would have greater access to more information and energy.

Another major factor that contributes to our lack of communication with the field is that we over identify with the mind. Majority of humans identify the contents of their mind as the highest authority. This is a natural process to go through; however, we are now at a level of consciousness growth, as far as humanity is concerned, where we are now invited more so than ever to move in the spaces beyond the mind. This is not to say that we discard the mind. No, we can still use the mind; it is very handy after all. However, we recognize that something else is there - something that is far more intelligent, peaceful and powerful than the mind could ever be. The more we go there, the more we can have access to its wonders.

After some time practicing the question and answer method and working some of these ideas and concepts into your world, it's likely that you will start to feel like the universe, or these higher non-physical beings are gently talking to you on a fairly regularly basis. It often comes through the feeling of strong intuition, strong feelings of energy, powerful dreams and even audible whispers in the ear. I also notice that sometimes the room around me begins to illuminate when the energy of this higher intelligence "joins in."

Its presence and guidance will never feel frightening or intimidating, for that is the case. It is not of the higher realms but more likely, the lower realms to which I would say steer away from as soon as possible. Instead, the presence of the field and the higher non-physical beings will always have a clear and warm feeling to them. Occasionally they may present an energy that has an "urgency" feeling to it, as a means to steer you away from immanent danger of some kind. However, it will always feel like it is being given in a supportive and friendly intention.

Overall, the more we open our context to include the field and the potential for higher, non-physical beings while also utilizing the questioning and answer method, the easier it will become to establish a meaningful relationship with the field. When this connection is established and nurtured, there will be an ongoing, friendly guidance that will permeate your experience and you will realize that you were never, and will never be truly alone.

Other ways to communicate with the field

1. When you go to sleep – what do I do with …?
If you are troubled or uncertain about something, when you go to bed that night, take a mmoment to think and ask with sincerity, "what do I do with ….?" Then, let it go, relax and go to sleep. When yu wake in the morning you will have a clear answer to the question you asked the night before. If not, then repeat for a few more days. Expect the solution to arise in your mind's eye and it will.

2. Wait for the obviousness to reveal itself
The truth is obvious – we just cant see or detect it because we are full of clutter; mental, emotional and physical clutter. Therefore, sometimes we just need to wait a little so that the truth of it will reveal itself.

3. If it's not an "F" yes, it's a No!
If the answer or the plan or whatever it is doesn't jump out at you, and make you want to go "F" yes, then generally it's a no. Life is too short and energy too precious to waste on half yes's. There will always be an "F" yes to be found in every situation.

4. Ceremony
Ceremonies can be very powerful for triggering changes in our state of consciousness. Ceremony also provide us with a dedicated time and space to focus our attention on the sacred.

Troubleshooting – How and Why Asking and Receiving Can Become Inaccurate

Methods to be more receptive
Awareness of body sensation will help anyone become more aware of the feelings and energy moving through their body and therefore make it much easier to test. Those people whose minds and bodies are "disconnected" often have a more difficult time with these types of practices. It's what I call a yin-yang split. The mind is not grounded in the body, so it's harder to utilize the body as a testing tool.

However, in saying that, the sway test has provided clear results on 99% of the people I have taught it. It has been by far the most accurate and clear testing method of the energy field I have witnessed and experienced over the last eight years.

The other thing I really like about it is that each individual can test themselves without involving another person. Therefore, the sway test encourages self-empowerment and self-discovery without the need for another person to be present.

Of course, sometimes having another person present, especially one who is well experienced with the technique and how to apply it therapeutically, is of great benefit. It is not always required but depends on where the tester is in their journey and what they are testing on.

Other suggestions for becoming more receptive are any practice or life attitude that brings the person more to the present time and therefore less engaged in mentalization. Meditation, letting go, breath awareness, yoga, tai-chi, qigong, martial arts, etc., are all helpful in practicing present moment awareness.

Diet can also play a role too through the use of pharmaceutical and non-pharmaceutical drugs. Anything that acts to dull the nervous system and one's mental sharpness can impede one's capacity to feel and notice the results from the testing. So this includes excessive use of alcohol, painkillers, and anti-anxiety medications. (If you are prescribed such medications, please speak with your medical doctor before any adjustments.)

Connecting with a Guide
It can be helpful for some people to work with a higher, non-physical light being. It does require a bit of groundwork and contextual reframing to be open to such an idea. As I am not an expert in creating such a context or pathway to this method, I cannot offer further guidance. However, there are a number of great authors and teachers out there that do provide a very safe, supportive and effective means to connecting with spirit guides. The book, *Opening to Channel* by Sanaya Roman and Duane Parker is an excellent book and great introduction into channeling.

The darker arts commonly associated with the occult is best to steer clear of. Human beings are not well equipped to deal with the forces and beings in the darker realms. It is not to say they don't exist, yet to play with, entertain or even invite these darker forces into our world is never a good idea. In terms of the energy field of the human being when it's exposed to occult symbolism and practices – it simply becomes weakened, therefore making our energy field much more susceptible to these darker beings.

Therefore, whenever engaging in working with energy beings, always make it a priority to be mentored and guided by an experienced practitioner with whom you have verified as working only with the higher beings of light.

Before you Test
As mentioned previously, you have to check yourself to make sure that you're "clear and devoid of bias." Essentially, this is about putting yourself into your higher self for the test.

If you test when you are unclear, intoxicated, feeling exhausted and are attached to an outcome, the test will not be clear and therefore, this is not a good time to carry out the test.

If such a condition or situation is present, try "switching on" using the various methods mentioned already in this book. Or, have a rest and get some sleep. When you wake up, you will have another opportunity to test again.

On energy testing and being "psychic"
This approach to asking the universe anything is, if you like, a kind of enhanced psychic perception.

While many of us do not have the perceptive abilities to experience visions and voices from the higher realms, we do, however, have the capacity to access the information in those realms via methods such as the ones explored in this book.

While many psychics and sensitive people do have access to higher realms of spirit, some also have access and practice with the lower realms of demonic entities. I personally do not encourage working with any lower realms in any circumstances, and the good news is that the method I explained in this book is only possible when using this method to access the higher realms of spirit. If we were to attempt to use it for accessing the lower realms, the information would simply come back unclear and unreliable, thus leading us to abandon any results. The only way to attain clear and reliable results is to work with the higher realms of spiritual truth, and this method is automatically set up to behave in this way. Therefore, following the guidelines in this book, there is no threat or possibility of going astray with this method.

Over time working with the sway testing method and establishing a sincere connection with the field, you will naturally become more acute and receptive to information and energy. It fortifies and fine-tunes our ability to be intuitive and for some, they may have more of their psychic space activated. The field is all intelligent and loving, so it will not drop or reveal things to us that we are not ready or able to work with. In other words, it will not make us "crazy". In fact, the opposite is true; it will bring us closer to states of peace, contentment, awe and humility. This comes about not because of an overload of information, but through a way of experiencing the vast beauty of the universe itself – with such revelation, one cannot but move into a space of pure humility and awe.

Conclusion

Overall, once the individual has awoken to the potential of the infinite field which surrounds and moves through us, we come to realize that all information is indeed available. It is through testing methods such as the "sway" test or the "sensing the heart" method that helps us establish a connection to the infinite power and intelligence of the field.

You may have also noticed that some questions are simply not appropriate or necessary for they do not inspire or contribute to the growth and development of the individual and the whole. To try and use these methods to predict lottery numbers or clarify gossip or trivialities will not work. See for yourself.

A natural re-contextualization occurs whenever we talk about or contemplate a power greater than our individual ego identity. It tends to expand in a way that allows more space for new insights and realizations to filter in.

The process of insight and realization, therefore, is not one of effort, or struggle, but simply due to the opening up of the heart and the reframing of the context in which we choose to live.

From here, it is worth continuing to explore and practice the questioning and answer methods explained in this book. It is natural for some people to take to the task wholeheartedly and practice it on everything, many times a day. This is a great and rapid way to becoming more familiar with it and start developing a more powerful relationship with the field. However, others may not be so enthusiastic to practice so readily, and that is ok, too.

The main thing is to practice checking in, "Is this true" or "does this feel true?" When you become good at this "checking in", the answer will present itself easily and readily. The main benefit from such a process is the avoidance of spending your precious time and energy engaged in the nonsense of the world which only acts to further confuse and distract us.

If you feel inspired to share these ideas and these testing methods with others, then please feel free to do so. The more people that are introduced and are practicing methods such as these ones, the more clarity is available to all of us. However, before sharing it is important that you feel established in the understanding and the practice yourself first so as not to add confusion or doubt.

There is no shortage of nonsense in our world, and the mind has a tendency to steer more towards it rather than away simply due to its glamorous, superficial appearance. However, when we start tasting the truth and clarity of deeper truths, it becomes obvious how distasteful nonsense really is. As soon as nonsense is detected, it is best to steer away. It is better to walk alone in truth than be surrounded by 100s who are caught in delusion.

The greatest gift we can offer the world is to simply align with higher truths, virtuous values and gain greater clarity. Only when this is in place will our thoughts, words and deeds be of some benefit to the world due to their alignment with the higher field. Those who have no connection to truth and clarity may speak fine words, yet the essence of those words are riddled with doubt and confusion.

Therefore, all that we really need to do is to make an effort to put ourselves in the flowing universal stream of truth and clarity. It is not a mind space but a deep, loving heart and energetic space. When we get established there, everything tends to work itself out without struggle or strain.

~ May All Beings Be Happy ~

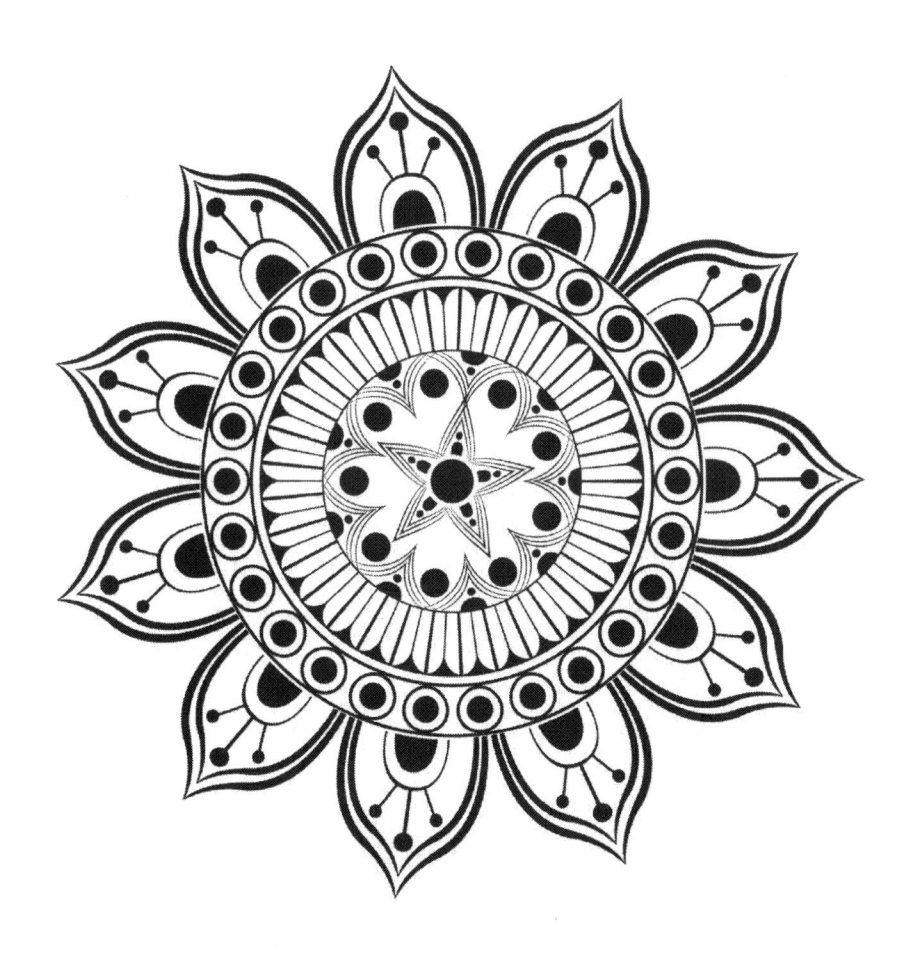

Can I ask you for a favor?

I hope you enjoyed the book and got something valuable from it. If so, could you please leave a review for me on Amazon?

I appreciate all of your feedback.

Each review also helps these ideas reach more people.

Thank you!
Hari Om!
~ Michael Hetherington

Sign up for the author's New Releases mailing list and **get a free copy** of *The Yin & Yang Lifestyle Guide*

Visit here ~
www.michaelhetherington.com.au/freebook

Other Titles by Author:

The Art of Self Muscle Testing
Learn how to access the human energy field for information

The Art of Self Adjusting
Learn how to stretch and make adjustments to the spine

EFT Through the Chakras
Work with EFT to clear the Chakras one by one

The Complete Book of Oriental Yoga
A journey into the 5 elements and yoga for the seasons

How to Do Restorative Yoga
Learn the art of a gentle yoga practice for deep relaxation

Increasing Internal Energy
Building energy from within to enhance daily life and strengthen our yoga practice

The greatest sin is to think yourself weak.

~ Swami Vivakananda

Made in the USA
San Bernardino, CA
04 November 2017